Legal Notice

This book is © 2022 Muhammad Sani. All Rights Reserved. Unauthorized Reproduction is Strictly Prohibited.

The information contained in this publication is for general information purposes only. While we endeavour to keep the information up-to-date and correct, we make no representations or warranties of any kind, express or implied, about the completeness, accuracy, reliability, suitability or availability with respect to the publication or the information, products, services, or related graphics contained in this publication for any purpose. Any reliance you, the reader place on such information is therefore strictly at your own risk. In no event will we be liable for any loss or damage including but not limited to; indirect or consequential loss or damage, or any loss or damage whatsoever arising from loss of data or profits stemming from or in connection with the use of this publication. We cannot guarantee results as results will differ from person to person and will depend on the effort taken. You are taking the decision to try this method, and there are no guarantees to your success.

No part of this eBook may be reproduced, copied or transmitted by any means – electronic or hard copy, including photocopying and recording - without expressly written and signed permission from the author. Violations of this copyright will be enforced to the fullest extent of the law.

Table Of Contents

Introduction

Chapter 1: Why Do I Gain Weight

- The Major Causes Of Weight Gain
- Should I Go On A Diet?
- Choosing The Right Diet Plan
- How Diets Work
- Industry Secrets

Chapter 2: What Do I Do Now?

- Stepping Out Of Your Comfort Zone
- Who to Approach When You Want to Lose Weight
- Persisting Through Failure

- Buddy System

- Why Maintaining a Daily Schedule is Critical

Chapter 3: Healthy Nutrition And Its Benefits

- Calories In – Calories Out

- Clean Eating

- Reducing Your Portions

- Water Is Your Best Friend

Chapter 4: The Importance Of Exercise

- Exercising

- The 3 Main Types Of Exercise

- Finding Exercises To Be Done At Home

Chapter 5: Living The Healthy Lifestyle

- The Healthy Lifestyle
- The Secrets of Staying Healthy
- The Advantages of Staying Healthy

Conclusion: Ready, Set, Go!

Introduction

Is this year finally the time you are going to say "Enough Is Enough"?
I am ready to start on a path to a healthier me, I'm NOT going to make any more excuses and I am going to make a change by shedding some of those extra pounds...No matter what!!!

If it is then get ready to...

DROP THE FAT AND CHANGE YOUR LIFE!

Today, it is simple to fall prey to promises of quick weight loss made by some diet plans, "magic diet pills," and other "wonder weight loss regimens." But in all honesty, it is a bunch of nonsense.

Before you choose your course of action, there are a few fundamental truths you should be aware of.

First of all, be aware that there is NO magic cure for weight loss.

While it is possible to lose a lot of weight by following a fad diet or other very restrictive eating plan, the major issue with doing so is the harm it causes to your health because it essentially deprives you of vital nutrients.

These diets may result in weak immunity, brittle bones, and overall worsening of health than before. More significant, however, is the issue that, if no lifestyle adjustments are made, the moment you stop depriving yourself while on a crash diet, you are very likely to go back to your old eating and exercising routines, which causes the dreaded Yo-Yo phenomenon.

According to studies, most overweight individuals who crash diet end up in considerably worse health than those who maintain their former weight are those who quickly gain back the weight they lost.

The question then becomes, "How can I lose weight?" And how can I improve my life and the lives of my family members?

The short answer is that this book is all about tried-and-true dietary and exercise recommendations because there is no such thing as a miracle.

This book's objective is to help the many regular people who are frantically trying to alter their lives—and the lives of their families—now and finally decide to lead healthier, happier, and more satisfying lives. This book will help, assist, and supply you with all the components you need to attain your goals and aspirations if you decide to make a commitment to lose weight and keep it off.

The time has come to decide to CHANGE YOUR LIFE AND LOSE THE FAT...FOREVER

Chapter 1

Why Do I Gain Weight?

It sure is challenging to maintain an active lifestyle and consume a healthy, balanced diet given the pace of our modern lives, the advent of technology, and the conveniences of fast food. But even with a busy lifestyle, it can be done if you know how to do it.

In this first section of the book we are going to look at:

- All the reasons why we gain weight,
- The people we need to talk to when we decide we are ready to lose the weight,
- Why keeping yourself on a schedule actually helps you to lose the weight,
- Weight loss secrets,
- Plus many other subjects that will help you to learn how to finally take the weight off and keep it off once and for all

The Major Causes Of Weight Gain

We consume more calories each day than our bodies require, and the extra is stored as fat. Because of the way our bodies are built, they can be ready for times when getting food was difficult by storing extra calories during times of abundance.
in a fatty form. Now, given how simple it is to obtain food, many individuals have a tendency to overeat, which is a serious issue that leads to a large number of people becoming overweight or obese..

- **Genetics play a factor as well by setting basic parameters on the metabolic efficiency of your body.** People who are obese frequently have extremely efficient metabolisms, which means that their bodies require fewer calories per day to function than those of others, and they store the extra calories as fat. Additionally, if both

of your parents are fat, your risk of developing the disease is significantly higher.

- **Your metabolic rate.** Your metabolic rate

is affected by your level of activity in addition to your genes. After we reach our mid-twenties, it is said that we lose roughly 10% of our metabolic rate every ten years. However, I believe that our level of activity has more to do with this than simply our age. Because muscle tissue is metabolically active but fat is not, the more active we are, the more muscle mass we may preserve or even increase, and as a result, the more fit we are. As we lose muscle mass, however, we are considerably more prone to acquire weight if we maintain a largely sedentary lifestyle.

- **Eating patterns.** People's eating habits make a huge difference in determining their weight. When foods high in fat or sugars are favoured, this of course can cause much weight gain. Also, how you serve the food, i.e. do you put the portions on everyone's plate or do you bring it all to the table and serve it the food family style where everyone can take as much as they want? Portion size is one of the main reasons people eat too much. Also, how have you learned to eat? If you are a fast eater, you may not even realize the cues your stomach gives you that it is full.

• **Larger portion sizes.** Over time, larger portions of food have become the norm, especially at many restaurants. Weight has also gone up because of this.

• **Exercise or the lack thereof.** A healthy lifestyle and maintaining a healthy weight both depend on exercise. When you exercise, especially when strength training is a part of your routine, you increase your metabolism, build muscle, and help the body burn more fat. Your weight will decrease as a result, and you'll appear leaner and firmer due to the fact that muscle takes up less space than fat. Strength training also improves bone density, aids in digestion, lowers blood pressure, cholesterol, and triglyceride levels, and lowers the risk of unintentional injury.

As you can see, diet and exercise are the two main factors that affect your health and weight, even if your genes make it easier for you to gain weight than other people. To reach and maintain a healthy weight, regular exercise is crucial. What you eat, how you eat, and how much you eat are also important factors.

Control your intake. The majority of people frequently underestimate how much they are eating due to this factor. Generally, you should only eat a portion of food the size of your fist at a time because that is also the size of your stomach.

You will be able to eat less and won't feel hungry in the beginning stages of developing this habit if you eat several small meals throughout the day as opposed to two or three large ones. Never skipping breakfast is another crucial rule because it sets your metabolism for the day. Your body will enter defence mode and store more fat if you skip breakfast because it will believe you are starving.

If you have a habit of eating quickly, try slowing down your eating as well. By doing this, you will be able to tell when you've had enough without stuffing yourself. Once you've done that, you can be certain that you've consumed too much food. When we are finished eating, we should actually feel

about a 5 on a scale of 1 to 10, in the middle of the range.
It takes some practice, but you can learn this trick and you will feel so much better knowing you did not stuff yourself to the maximum capacity.
Another thing to watch of course is your intake of fatty and sugary foods. We all need nutrients, including healthy fats, to keep us balanced, but eating a lot of junk food and sugary drinks will attribute greatly to us gaining more weight. Processed foods don't generally have a lot of nutrients in them, or any at all, and they are high in salt, sugar, and unhealthy fats.

In today's busy lifestyles, we may not realize how often we are eating these foods. If you are one who is always ordering out for work, or going out to dinner as well, this is not going to keep you healthy because you do not have the control as to what is being put

in your food (except special ordering at a restaurant) and it is much harder to make sure you are eating the right kinds of things and getting all of your nutrients. Going out to eat is fine every once in a while, but be sensible in what you are choosing, and you don't have to clear your plate of the large servings you will most likely be given.

Should I Go On A Diet?

Most individuals think of dieting when they want to lose weight. Finding a fad diet that is undoubtedly popular at the moment and trying to adhere to all of its bizarre rules and recipes, such as lemon juice, cayenne pepper, and maple syrup, are frequent examples of what this entails. But who actually likes these things? Do you enjoy avoiding entire food groups like carbohydrates or consuming bizarre mixtures that just don't taste good or fill you up?
Nobody probably does, to be honest. Yes, there are other diets that are very effective. If you decide that going on a diet is what you want to do, it is very advisable to research the various diets available so that you can find a reasonable, sensible diet that won't harm you or drive you crazy with hunger and make you fail in the end.

Choosing the Right Diet Plan

When you are ready to choose your diet or eating plan, there are certain things that you must take into consideration to make sure that you are picking one that will help you to attain the weight loss goals you have and to make sure you are staying healthy. Some diets, as we mentioned, do not contain the right balance of nutrition that your body's needs, and can therefore make you sick, and won't help you to lose weight properly.

When selecting the ideal diet, bear the following considerations in mind:

• **Realistic Expectations:** You need to understand that reducing

weight is a process that requires patience. The amount of weight you need to shed to reach your ideal weight will determine how long it will take you to reach your objectives. You shouldn't commit to a crash diet that guarantees you'll drop a lot of weight quickly because doing so will probably be dangerous and extremely harmful for you. You should lose about 1-2 pounds a week to maintain a healthy weight reduction after the first two or three weeks, when weight loss is quick due to water loss.

• **The Right Nutrition:** Make sure to carefully review any diet plans you are thinking about and see what they recommend or allow you to eat. You are probably looking at a safe plan if it features a balanced diet that includes the proper proportions of foods from the major food groups. Any fad diet that forces you to eliminate entire food groups, starve yourself, or consume bizarre concoctions is unsafe. Additionally, be sure you are getting no more than 30% of your daily calories from fat and that you are getting the correct mix of protein, carbs, and fibre.

• **The Right Fit For You...or Not?** Make sure the diet you choose would suit your lifestyle and the one you are researching while you are doing your research. Look for a plan that offers convenience in addition to healthy options if you are a very busy individual who spends little time at home. If you end up making a decision that prevents you from following through on your plan for any reason, you will fail and are likely to revert to your old habits while feeling worse than before.

- **Calorie Level:** Make sure you are consuming enough calories according to the strategy you select. In essence, you want to reduce your calorie intake to the point where you can lose those 1-2 pounds each week. You must weigh all of this against yourself and your level of activity because everyone differs in how many calories they require daily. depending on how active they are and their weight. You might want to work with a trained health professional to help you decide which is best for you.

How Diets Work

It's easy to lose weight—just burn off more calories than you consume.

It is a requirement for us to eat. Our bodies will break down the food we eat, keeping only what is necessary, and discarding the remainder. As we go about our daily lives, our bodies use the calories and nutrients from meals as fuel to get everything done. However, because our body only requires a set number of calories for this, any extra calories are stored as fat in our bodies.

Our body has the limitation that we are unable to instruct it to stop accumulating calories. No matter how much fat you already have in your body, all more calories will be turned into fat. Most people always eat more than they should, consuming additional calories that cause us to gain weight.

"So in essence a diet is supposed to help you lose those extra calories"

A Diet is a way of eating where you would limit your calorie intake. Not all diets involve cutting back on calories. You can consume continual food as long as it is low in calories as the goal is to eat less calories. Therefore, if you compare foods like fruit or vegetables to other foods like meat, they have fewer calories per serving.

You will eat significantly less when on a diet. As a result, you would have increased hunger throughout the day and increased dissatisfaction after eating. Since you are aiming to consume less calories, it cannot be prevented. Do not confuse missing meals or going without food. These will simply make your diet problems worse.

A healthy diet should include strategies for psychologically and

physically squelching hunger. Before beginning a diet, you must always psychologically prepare yourself. This is to make sure that you can adhere to the diet plan throughout and accomplish your objective. Diet plans will also provide substitute snacks for you to eat in order to save your desires.

Never assume that a diet would consist of nothing but water and veggies for the entire day. In fact, diet encourages eating a variety of foods. You should not overlook the other nutrients in order to merely reduce your calorie intake.

Therefore, you would also be avoiding their nutrients if you avoid a particular type of food. The diet plan will therefore outline alternate foods that you can eat to make up for the nutrients that are missing. Typically, these items are avoided but not outright prohibited. Therefore, you can occasionally eat them in little portions.

A healthy diet also supports your body's natural metabolism. Everybody has a different rate of metabolism. A person who has a faster metabolism can burn more calories each day. People with slow metabolic rates might better utilize their energy with the right eating plan.

such as eating a healthy breakfast to kick-start the metabolism, a filling lunch to keep you going, and a smaller dinner because you burn fewer calories at night. This will guarantee that you consume adequate calories throughout the day.

Rule of Thumb

One of the key components to sticking to a diet plan is discipline. It can take months or even years to lose weight through a proper diet and get to your ideal weight. Extreme diets that encourage rapid weight loss can develop into yo-yo dieting. Yo-yo dieting is the practice of losing weight while adhering to a diet, only to gain it all back and then some.

This occurs as a result of the extreme nature of the diet he followed, which severely restricted his food intake and prohibited many food groups. He can't follow all these diets, so he caves and eats more. Or it might be the result of a lack of discipline once the desired weight has been reached. This is typically what happens when you follow an extremely high-calorie diet.

Dieters are therefore advised to start slowly with their diets because most people will give up midway through and it will take months to see significant results. It is difficult to break a habit that you've had for a long time. For this reason, maintaining a diet requires a lot of self-control, willpower, and determination.

At first, breaking a habit is challenging. For the first month, you must adhere to your daily diet plan. The foundation will be laid by this. It is believed that you have formed a new habit after 30 days.

Everyone can diet together. I sincerely advise you to enlist the aid of a friend or perhaps to diet together. You can also gradually witness the results in each other by having someone by your side to support you. When you feel that the diet is not working for you, it also helps to have a confidant.

Consider a few diets that might be similar to the one you are already on when choosing a diet to follow. This will broaden the diet. Your willpower will suffer in the future if you continue to eat the same diet that you detest.

You might even give up on your diet as a result of this. You can therefore select a diet plan that you'll appreciate and not get bored watching what you eat by varying your diet.

You can change your diet plan on a weekly or monthly basis to keep it current.

Just keep in mind that just because you missed one of your diet meals, the remainder of the day does not have to be wrecked and you should still stick to your diet plan. Just carry on with your day as if you had never cheated on your diet. This eventually results in long-term weight loss or management.

Industry Secrets

The weight loss business is keeping a number of facts from you and doesn't want you to know them. They are selling fads, devices, and pills to people who are desperate to lose weight, and their business is booming as a result. Unfortunately, people's wallets are typically the only item that is growing lighter. Only a small portion of those who adopt one of these strategies actually succeed in losing weight and keeping it off. Many of these methods are ineffective..

Some of These Industry Secrets Include:

- **Most weight loss product ads deceive the buyer.** A majority of the weight loss products you hear about on the radio and see on infomercials don't even do what they claim to. Even so, consumers are lured into buying these products with promises like "Lose the weight and keep it off", "Eat whatever you want" and "no diet or exercise required". Basically, if it sounds too good to be true, it most likely is.

- **Just because they say it's "scientifically proven" or "doctor-endorsed" doesn't mean it works.** These claims are typical as well, but they never tell you anything about where the studies were made or by who so that you can check out the validity for yourself.
And what does it really mean anyway? Often these so-called health professionals have a financial interest in the product, and probably did not review the scientific evidence. If it was reviewed, they may not have even used acceptable review standards. Why would you want to risk your health on such a thing?

- **Just because the government allows a product to be on the market does not mean it is safe for consumers or that it does what it claims.** There is a huge misconception that the government would not allow a product on the market if it could

potentially be harmful to you. People tend to think that the government has to pre-approve them first, but many times that is not the case.

- **Natural or herbal products are not always guaranteed to be safe**

It makes it much more challenging the next time you try to lose weight. The belief that a product must be safe just because it contains natural ingredients is another common misconception. However, corporations are able to release their items onto the market up until the FDA obtains proof that a product is hazardous.

You shouldn't believe everything you hear since it may not be true. You should avoid items that make grandiose claims because there are many out there that just do not live up to their claims.

Likewise, don't believe the claims made by fad diets. Anything that calls for abrupt and drastic adjustments to your dietary habits is very challenging to maintain over time. They'll start you on a rapid weight-loss cycle, which is always followed by a period during which, in some cases, you'll gain all the weight you lost plus some once your regular eating patterns restart. And It. These diets have no positive effects on health, and do you really believe that there would be a demand for new ones if they did?

Additionally, you shouldn't rely on the money-back guarantee. The likelihood of getting your money back is about equal to the likelihood that the product will live up to its promises.

Additionally, there isn't a miracle cure or quick fix that will enable you to ultimately reduce weight. If a product makes such claims, you can almost certainly rest assured that it won't be true.

Chapter 2

What Do I Do Now?

You must be dedicated to any diet in order to succeed at it. The only way to succeed is to have the appropriate mindset. Before you can go on to the next phase of your diet, you must first prepare yourself by understanding what stage you are in. It may not be seen, yet it is nonetheless present.

The First stage is pre-contemplation. You don't think of yourself as overweight. You don't feel like altering who you are. You won't ask for aid unless there is a lot of strain. But if that happened, you wouldn't give in; you'd just give up, feeling defeated by your own situation.

Second is contemplation. This is the point at which you admit that you have a weight problem and begin to plan a remedy. However, you are unwilling to implement that remedy. You wouldn't do anything but mull it over, knowing what you should do to change things but never being prepared to act. You will put off implementing the solution.

Third is preparation. You've finally made up your mind to address your weight issue. You stop dwelling on your issue and start identifying the answer. Additionally, you might begin to see a time in the future when you are thinner and feel much better. However, you haven't totally overcome your issues just yet. You would still have second thoughts about the solution as it requires you to change your lifestyle.

Fourth is action. You start to take action in losing weight. You would start choosing the food you eat and do some form of exercise every day. It is the first step in achieving your targeted goal.

You should always set goals when losing weight. If you don't set your goals, then it's very possible that your whole dieting plan might not go the way you imagine it.

"If you don't plan, you plan to fail,"

they say.

List the following:

- **What is your current situation right now**? List all your eating habits, food preferences, everything that could affect your weight loss. Working out, etc

- **What is the reason you want to lose weight**? This could be an upcoming event, summer, or even for a certain special someone. List the single BIGGEST reason you can think of.

- **What are the benefits you get from your weight loss**? List AS MANY as you can. It can be health, better energy, admired by partner, etc. This should be your main motivator.

- **Your Goal. "I want to lose XX lbs of weight in XX days"** - Write this in bold and make it really sink in. I would personally say that setting a goal of more than 10 lbs per 2 weeks is not realistic, especially if this is your first attempt at a goal like this. Be realistic. You must write "I want" not "I wish"

Write everything down and look at that paper every day. Put it in a place where you can see it. Once you see it every day, you will constantly be reminded of WHY you do this and what the benefits are.

BE PERSISTENT ONCE YOU TAKE ACTION BECAUSE IT'S NOT GOING TO BE EASY

STEPPING OUT OF YOUR COMFORT ZONE.

If you see yourself making excuses rather than STARTING a diet that is effective, you should think about why you don't really want to lose weight. You must be able to step out of your comfort zone and as Nike's famous slogan goes **JUST DO IT!**

Maintenance would be the last stage. You must maintain the momentum you had throughout the action stage. If you ever stop being dedicated or supportive, you will revert to any of the earlier stages.

The final step of your diet plan is therefore the most crucial because you need to maintain your dedication over an extended length of time. There are various strategies you can employ to maintain your commitment. Make a list of your initial motivations for doing this before anything else. To keep your focus on your goals, review the list every day. Avoid thinking anything unfavourable. Never use words like "never" or "depriving" in your vocabulary. You are only enjoying sweets "sometimes and in moderation" rather than "never." As a result, the word "starved" might be changed to "choosing" as you have decided to forego chocolate cakes.

Imagine in your mind's eye a slimmer version of yourself accomplishing all the things you have always desired. Your determination to stick with this plan and be determined to succeed will be boosted by this visualization. Every morning and any moment during the day that you feel your

dedication waning, use this visualization.
Who to Approach When You Want to Lose Weight

Now that you've decided you want to lose weight, you should include some other people in your weight loss journey. These people can help you with many aspects, including choosing your diet plan, setting your goals and encouraging you along the way.

• **A Therapist:** Even though they are aware of how detrimental their overeating is for them, some people just can't manage to control it. Many of these individuals overeat due to emotional factors like loneliness or dissatisfaction and use food as a way to mask their hurt and other emotions.

People who do this should consult a therapist or other experts with training in this area so they can receive the right support. In extremely extreme circumstances, it may be necessary to check themselves into a specialized clinic created for this reason in order to closely monitor their diet and activity.

• **A Dietician:** Since a medical license is typically needed before becoming a dietician in most states and nations, they will have a wide range of knowledge that can assist you in understanding your body and preparing a diet that will meet your specific needs.

Their objective is to encourage you to eat healthier so that you can reduce your weight. Because fad diets may not be nutritionally sound for you, dieticians are distinguished from those who advocate them. A dietician can also help you balance your consumption of the various food groups you should be consuming from and determine how many calories you need to consume each day.

• **A Physical Trainer:** Most people have never been taught how to exercise correctly. A physical trainer will make sure that you do, will encourage you to achieve your goals, and can even assist in the goal-setting process. They will supervise your gym workout and provide you with both cardio and strength-based activities to do. A personal trainer's main objective is to help you get fit, and they also provide you advice on how to do it right for yourself. Each person has unique demands, and a personal trainer can modify your exercise regimen to best suit you. As you begin to acquire more muscular tone to support your new muscles during the weight loss process, your physical trainer and dietarian may advise you to switch up your food and exercise regimen.

• **Friends and Family:** You might wish to share your weight loss journey with friends and family at the beginning so they can offer encouragement. People you know and trust supporting you in any attempt is usually helpful.

Even better, have a buddy or your spouse hold you responsible to them, prevent you from sneaking extra snacks or treats, or encourage you to stick with your exercise routine. If you have someone by your side (even over the phone if they are far away), who will support you and push you when you start to falter, you will probably be more successful in the long run. Once you accomplish your ultimate objective (or possibly several smaller ones along the way), you can enjoy a celebration with your loved ones.

Persisting Through Failure

If you want to commit to losing weight, then you need to be able to persist through failure. Everyone who has accomplished something of note has struggled with failure at one or more points in their ascent. The difference is they didn't quit when it got tough, persisted through it and learned a lesson.

"When the going gets tough, the tough get going"

The two main strategies for handling failure are those. Keep trying and picking things up.
Don't worry if you stray from your diet or skip a day of exercise. Don't allow it to stop

you. Get it out of your head. Consider all of your good days rather than just one mistake. The more healthier lifestyle choices you make, the more good days you have; before you realize it, the bad days are few and far between. But the key is to persevere and get through the difficult times. Consider it a cheat day, then move on. This is how you persevere; it's okay to fail for a day, but don't allow it turn into a week, then a month.

To deal with failures, you must learn to accept them as a natural part of life.

The next step is to take lessons from your errors. It is frequently more effective to learn from your errors than from your accomplishments. When you fail, view it as a teaching moment. Just like in business, when you try something and fail, you learn what doesn't work. The same holds true for losing weight. If every time you drink, you fall off your new diet, perhaps you don't drink at all. Reschedule your workout if you find that you consistently skip it on Fridays due to a late work meeting.

> *"I have not failed. I've just found 10,000 ways that won't work."*
> *—Thomas A Edison*

Along with death and taxes, failure is a given in life. Even if you could, you wouldn't want to since you can't prevent it. Your failures and successes both teach you valuable lessons about life. Don't be afraid of failing; just keep trying and keep learning.

Buddy System

One of the best things you can do when you are trying to lose weight is to add some accountability to your routine. How do you do that?

The buddy system.

A fantastic motivation is having a friend with whom to attempt weight loss. When you actually tell someone about your weight loss objectives, you will feel more responsible for achieving them. They can also be useful because the person can understand your difficulties with weight loss. You can encourage one another by sharing both your victories and your setbacks.

A workout partner is invaluable if you exercise frequently. They can transform a dull jog or walk into a therapy session that also serves as exercise. Bringing a friend along for a hike in the wilderness is always more enjoyable! Having a friend is also beneficial if you enjoy weightlifting. You guys can push each other while also encouraging and helping each other out with things like spots on heavy lifts.
The sad truth is that you can probably find a weight loss buddy in your circle of friends today. Don't worry if you can't; you can always do it virtually online. You could collaborate with a Facebook friend who is trying to lose weight. chatting on Facebook and posting images of one's progress. Additionally, there are a ton of websites and forums devoted to virtually connecting weight loss partners.

The bottom line is that working with a friend can help with accountability, support, and motivation if you're trying to lose weight. Now go find your weight-loss partner!

Why Maintaining a Daily Schedule is Critical

Setting up a daily program for yourself is the next stage in preparing your weight reduction objectives. You must choose the optimal time of day for you to workout. For instance, getting up two hours earlier than usual is probably not a smart idea if you are not a morning person because you will likely miss many mornings.

Likewise, planning your workouts for after work is not a smart idea if your employment routinely requires you to work late into the evenings. Additionally, you can plan out your meals, including the times you eat each day and the contents of your meals. The best course of action is to plan them out for weeks at a time, make a list, and follow it, so that when you go shopping you won't be as tempted to make impulsive purchases or deviate from your diet.

• **Maintaining Your Balance:** You are more likely to keep to your goals if you write everything down in a notebook or other note-taking tool, such as a smart phone, provided you have a set plan to follow. However, if you do skip a workout or have an extra snack,

you can mark it and resolve to do better the following time.

• **Knowing Your Daily Activities:** If you know in advance when you should exercise or eat, you may plan your day accordingly. This prevents you from scheduling other activities around your workout times and causes you to skip those activities entirely. This is simple to accomplish, and if you do it frequently enough, you will soon miss more sessions until you entirely lose track of your fitness goals.

• **Lose More Weight:** You will most likely lose more weight overall if you stick to a timetable because you won't skip any sessions (or very, very few in the long run). You will find it much more difficult to maintain a consistent pace of weight reduction if you frequently switch between diets, skip workouts, or skip meals, which confuses your body's metabolism.

Chapter 3

Healthy Nutrition And Its Benefits

You may have heard a lot of people claim that eating a healthy diet is essential for maintaining a healthy body, but you should understand what healthy nutrition actually entails and why it is so crucial. Define nutrition first.

"Nutrition is the process of giving your body all the essential nutrients that will enable it to develop in a healthy and balanced manner.
This is the simplest description of nutrition, and it informs you that you must consume healthy foods that are rich in essential nutrients. While an unhealthy nutrition plan can weaken your body, make you ill, and prevent you from fighting off some mild ailments, a healthy nutrition plan can keep your body strong and healthy as well as help

it grow and repair itself.

Calories In - Calories Out

Most people who want to lose weight have experimented with a variety of diets, supplements, and/or plans. There are many different weight loss strategies that can be purchased. They're all making outrageous claims.
The harsh reality is that there are no magic pills, diets, or exercise equipment that will make weight vanish overnight. It all comes down to eating properly, maintaining good health, and consuming fewer calories than you expend.
That is the origin of the proverb "calories in, calories out." Make sure you expend more calories (out) than you take in (in).

This is a naive way of thinking, and a healthy diet involves more than just counting calories. We'll examine that in later chapters, but for now, let's focus on establishing a calorie deficit.
You'll need some basic information to track this. You must first determine how many

calories you naturally burn each day. It all comes down to things like weight and age.

Calculating the Number of Calories You Burn Daily

BMR calculation for men (kg)	BMR = 66.5 + (13.75 x weight in kg) + (5.003 x height in cm) − (6.755 x age in years)
BMR calculation for men (pounds)	BMR = 66 + (6.23 x weight in pounds) + (12.7 x height in inches) − (6.76 x age in years)
BMR calculation for women (kg)	BMR = 655.1 + (9.563 x weight in kg) + (1.850 x height in cm) − (4.676 x age in years)
BMR calculation for women (pounds)	BMR = 655 + (4.35 x weight in pounds) + (4.7 x height in inches) − (4.7 x age in years)

This formula will give you the basic calories you burn daily, just by breathing, heart pumping and etc... These are how many calories you burn if you didn't move all day (basal metabolic rate).

Once you have that number, you need to start tracking the calories you burn and the calories you consume. This can be tricky because it is a lot of information to keep track of.

There are websites that can help though:

http://caloriecount.about.com/

This is one of the more popular calorie counters out there since it is free. It will help you track what you eat, and what you expend.

You just have to enter the foods and activity you had for the day. It will even allow you to input your basal metabolic rate.

It is ideal if you can keep a daily caloric deficit, but that isn't always possible. Sometimes we slip and sometimes we indulge. If you can get a weekly caloric deficit that will still have you losing weight.

This isn't about starving yourself, or exercising until you are dead. It is all about being aware what you put in your body, and what you exert. Weight loss can be a struggle, but if you can manage your calories in and calories out - you can overcome!

Clean Eating

The fundamental weight reduction principle, calories in versus calories out, has already been discussed. It is a fundamental guideline since you still need to be cautious about where you are obtaining your calories from. It's probably not a good idea to have two corndogs every day in order to reduce your calorie intake.

Although the phrase "eating clean" lacks an official definition, in general it means:

"Eating natural, nutritious foods and staying away from processed foods and refined sweets."

While it may not always be practical to

consume only "clean" foods, if you are obtaining the majority of your calories from these foods, you are doing excellent. Fast food and junk food are automatically eliminated from your diet when you eat clean since you avoid processed foods. Don't worry if you consume some processed food; the goal is to consume as little of it as possible.

Here are some general clean eating tips:

- **Learn to read labels!** Read the nutritional information and ingredients of everything you buy.
- **Choose while grains when possible**. Whole wheat doesn't necessarily mean whole grain either! Look for bread, pasta and etc... that are made with 100% whole grains
- **Eat lots of fruits and vegetables**. They are great whole sources of clean calories
- **Prepare more of your own meals**, don't eat out as much or buy microwaveable type meals. These meals even when "healthy", can be loaded with things like sodium.

- **Choose lean meats when cooking**. Eating meat is fine and the protein will help build muscle and make you feel full. Chicken and fish are great meat choices.
- **Avoid processed meats like bologna or hot dogs.**
- **Replace junk food with unsalted or lightly salted whole nuts**.
- **Check out the internet for great clean recipes. Keep a list!**
- **Don't fret over falling off the wagon**, even grat yourself a cheat day now and then.
- **Eating clean while out can be tough but more restaurants are offering clean menu items**. A Salad can be a good choice, but if you are really hungry you might need to add some protein!
- **Start as soon as possible!**

A wonderful strategy to ensure that you are healthy overall and that you lose weight is to eat cleanly. You don't have to try to turn on a switch and make the change overnight, but it isn't always simple. Clean up your diet if you're serious about reducing weight and improving your health.

Reducing Your Portions!

Anyone trying to lose weight should think about portion control. Just ask anyone who has successfully shed pounds (and sustained it). Portion control will almost certainly be mentioned as one of the secrets to their success.

Portion Control: What Is It?
Understanding serving sizes and calorie counts is the first step in practicing portion control.

Realizing what constitutes a proper portion of food is one of the biggest challenges faced by overweight people. Realize what a serving size of your foods is before you sit down to a meal. While not scientific, the following list offers you an idea of some recommended portion sizes. If you have trouble losing weight, you might find that these portions are smaller than you anticipated:

- Vegetables or fruit is about the size of your fist.
- Pasta is about the size of one scoop of ice cream.
- Meat, fish, or poultry is the size of a deck of cards or the size of your palm (minus the fingers).
- Snacks such as pretzels and nuts are about the size of a cupped handful.
- Potato is the size of a computer mouse.
- Steamed rice is the size of a cupcake wrapper.
- Cheese is the size of a pair of dice or the size of your whole thumb (from the tip to the base).

I can attest that when I initially noticed the cheese serving size, it startled me. Online resources provide information on portions. Online resources can include considerably more detailed portion control instructions. You might need to weigh your food in order to get precise servings because some websites split it down by food weight. However, the list above is sufficient to give you a general notion.

Watch your portion sizes while you eat! One of the most important stages you'll take on your weight loss quest is figuring out how much food you actually need.

The key to losing weight is to spread meals out into smaller portions rather than consuming large meals all at once. It has been demonstrated that restricting your meals not only lowers your daily calorie consumption but also supports a constant metabolism. Consider eating 6-7 smaller meals spaced out throughout the day if you typically eat 2-3 large meals per day.

Instead than taking out what they need and putting the packet away, some people prefer to eat directly from the packet. An illustration of this would be eating potato chips straight out of a giant packet. In addition to not knowing how much you are eating, you frequently overeat in order to satisfy a hunger when all you need to do is put a small amount of the food you are eating into a bowl with a piece of fruit to get the right amount of food.

Now more than ever, huge packets are the norm. More products are being offered in bulk, and more meals are being served in supersized portions at restaurants for a small fee. Increased portions are a contributing element in the rising obesity rates. There is always a reason, yet people frequently prioritize fun over everything else, putting their health at danger. Because of this, restricting meals is a useful strategy for breaking undesirable behaviours.

Making changes requires discipline, and there's really no need for people to believe they should keep eating past the point of fullness. Always eat small portions; if you're still hungry, add a tiny bit more rather than piling food on your plate and attempting to finish it all. Giving yourself room to eat another small meal a few hours later and still feel well enough to squeeze in some exercise is a good balance that will produce better results than sitting around feeling stuffed and undoing your belt buckle.

By doing this, you can control your weight and watch it slowly start to drop. This wonderful feeling will encourage you to work a little harder as you grow more confident in your ability to control your body and resist giving in to cravings.

Water Is Your Best Friend

According to research, you should drink at least 8 glasses of water each day, but how much you actually need will depend on your weight. A man weighing 180 pounds would require 60 ounces of water per day, so you would need to divide your weight by 2.

So why is water recommended by experts and why is it seen to be so vital to living a healthy life?

First off, it helps to prevent dehydration, it maintains the kidneys

healthy by aiding in the removal of waste materials, and it also helps to enhance your metabolism, which aids in weight loss. But in addition to paying attention to what professionals advise, you should prioritize paying attention to your body. Naturally, you will drink water to rehydrate yourself when you are thirsty.

You should strive to develop the habit of routinely consuming water or, better yet, keeping a water bottle nearby depending on the type of work you do.

A water bottle is useful, especially on really hot days when sweating and water loss from the body mean that you will need to replenish yourself.

Water has a crucial role in our lives because of this. In addition to having no calories, it is also the best and healthiest way to quench your thirst. In the long run, you might think about replacing fruit drinks and sodas with water at all of your meals because it will help you consume fewer calories and you'll feel much better without the extra sugar that comes with the other drinks.

Chapter 4

The Importance Of Exercise

In this chapter, I will tell you about different types of exercises and their effects on different aspects of your life and health.

☐ Exercise to improve bone and muscle strength
☐ Flexibility increasing exercises
☐ Cardiovascular exercise
☐ Aerobics

Exercising

Dieting and exercise are complementary activities. If you only diet without exercising, you might not see any results at all because your diet isn't causing you to burn calories quickly enough. In addition, you would appear skinny and feeble as you lost your fat if you did manage to reduce weight without dieting. So while dieting, it is preferable to exercise to keep your body in shape. There are further justifications for exercising.

"A recent survey showed that seven out of ten adults do not exercise regularly and close to four out of ten are not physically active. If you do not exercise, then you will risk getting stroke, diabetes and heart disease. This has lead to death for about 300 000 people."

You should speak with a doctor before beginning an exercise program. Knowing your current physical condition will help you determine whether engaging in strenuous exercise may put you at risk for injuries. Start out cautiously when you initially start exercising. Start off with just 10 minutes, then increase it to 20 minutes, then 30 minutes, and so on over the course of several months. This will lessen the likelihood of damage and prevent your body from feeling overly sore after each workout.

Every day, you should engage in moderate cardiovascular activity for at least 30 minutes or more. It's okay to break up the 30 minutes into shorter, irregular bursts of activity. Do muscle-building exercises twice a week after that. This physical activity can be incorporated into your regular routine. Take the stairs rather than the elevator to get to the office; jog during lunch; or park further away from your place of employment, as examples.

Why not try to make your free time more active if you feel like this is too much of a work. Ask your family to go on a family bike trip, join a rock climbing club, or just take a stroll in the park every evening instead of staying home alone.

Choose exercises that you will love performing, find fulfilling, and make you feel accomplished. You'll be more motivated to exercise after a successful run. Make it simple for yourself to be active by choosing an activity that is more easily available so you won't lose motivation every time you want to exercise. Choose a form of exercise that is appropriate for your age and physical condition.

The 3 Main Types Of Exercise

You must first be aware that there are three main types of workout programs available, and each one offers a unique set of benefits for your physical well-being.

Exercise To Strengthen Bones And Muscles

Strength and resistance training are other names for these workouts. Most people mistake bodybuilding for exercises that increase strength and resistance, but you should be aware that bodybuilding is a different type of exercise where the person's main objective is to promote muscle growth. Your fat-burning and weight-control plan can include weightlifting and bodybuilding, but only to the extent that your body can do it

without experiencing any problems. Your entire body may be a wreck if you overdid this activity. I've witnessed individuals join gyms and engage in strenuous exercise simply by observing others do it. This is not the way to proceed; instead, speak with your trainer in person and inquire about the best workouts for your needs. You don't need to lift large weights if your weight is under control and you only need mild exercise to maintain a healthy system.

Exercises to Increase Flexibility

Your body needs to become more flexible if you frequently have pain in your arms, legs, lower back, neck, or other comparable areas of your body. This is referred to as the second sort of workout regimen. Increased resistance and easier adaptation to more challenging situations and postures are both benefits of flexibility. Daily living requires you to adopt various postures. For instance, if you work in an office, you may occasionally be forced to sit in an uncomfortable chair or you may be given tasks that require intense concentration on a computer screen and prevent you from using a chair to rest your back. Lack of flexibility will cause issues in these circumstances, but regular flexibility exercises, which shouldn't take more than 10-15 minutes, will improve your flexibility and help you feel better and more active.

Heart-Healthy Exercise

Cardio means heart, vascular means blood vessels, and this entire term suggests that these exercises improve the functionality of your lungs, increase the efficiency with which you use oxygen, and address any potential cardiac issues you may have. These short-duration exercises should be properly learned from your trainer or doctor. People who already have a heart condition frequently engage in these exercises to prevent further issues.

Finding Exercises To Be Done At Home

Workout fanatics are moving their workouts

from gyms to their homes, which is a significant shift in their behavior. The skyrocketing membership costs and legally enforceable contracts are the causes. They have thus begun to choose home fitness regimens.

Finding exercises to do at home is not a difficult task; rather, it is a far more practical choice. Numerous excellent cardio exercises are available that people may perform for little to no cost. Depending on the desired activity, the main investment is in a nice pair of walking, jogging, or aerobic shoes. A jumping rope is also an excellent addition for home skipping since it gives users other aerobic exercise options, some of which include rapid work interval training. It can be done while watching TV or possibly with music playing in the background. Jumping should be done as quickly as possible for 30 to 1 minute, followed by a short break before starting again. You can always do it during the commercial breaks as you watch the rest of the program when your body is calming down. The market for videos and DVDs is oversaturated with

Workout, aerobics, and yoga CDs and DVDs are available for purchase if you want to start an effective home exercise program for fitness.
This gives consumers more options in the event that jogging or walking gets boring or if the weather prevents running outside. When done with a companion, walking and running can actually become more exciting, as long as no chit-chat or gossip sessions take precedence over your workout regimen.

The daily exercise routine can be changed by changing the surface where you run or stroll. To maintain your fitness, keep in mind that enjoyment is crucial if you want to see changes in your health and physical appearance. In addition, age does factor into the type of exercise you choose. An adult may be able to build muscle and lose weight using specific equipment, but an elderly person may not just

get the same results.

Same outcomes from the same program. It is solely due to performance quality and not because expensive and comparable machines were used. Thu, it's advised that you always pick a fitness routine that works with your body, age, and needs while taking into account the various health restrictions that aging brings with it.

Home workouts that you can carry out

Leaving you with no excuses of not finding the right type of exercises that you can do at home, here is a list of the appropriate home fitness based program exercises for you-

☐ These exercises can be performed by using easy drills at home and employing minimal
equipments which you can get from around your house.

☐ For upper body you can do chair dips, lateral raises, push-ups, chin ups and bent over row. For core exercises you can do dead lift, sit ups and Side Bridge.

☐ For lower body you can opt for step ups, wall squat, bucket squats and lunges.

You must warm up for a minimum of five minutes before beginning these exercises by jogging, taking a fast walk around the block, or skipping on the spot. Depending on your endurance level and the exercises' requirements, you must execute various sets of the aforementioned exercises. Additionally, taking breaks is also important. Combining two workouts that work different muscle groups and switching between the two can provide each muscle group a rest between exercises.

Perform these exercises at least three times a week for the best results, allowing at least a day between sets to allow for adequate recovery. To improve your fitness growth, you must always work to increase the intensity or load. Once your fitness level increases, you may perform this exercise without much difficulty and go on to a better program. Find more items to utilize for at-home exercise by using your creativity.

For squats and step-ups, you can use

buckets that have been filled with however much water you like.

Milk bottles may be made to weigh the same as a 2 kg weight by filling them with 2 litres of water.
for bent-over rows, bicep curls, and overhead triceps extensions.

Lunges, step-ups, and squats can be performed using shopping bags and backpacks loaded with objects. For push ups, bench press, lateral raises, and front rises, it is permissible to use bricks that have been broken in half in cases of lighter weight.

Next follow the traditional exercise modalities that are a part of yoga asana. Many people engage in these exercises not just to reduce mental stress but also to become and maintain physical fitness. When it comes to their bodies, yoga has done wonders for every renowned celebrity today, including household names like Jennifer Aniston and Drew Barrymore, giving them the kind of figure every girl dreams of having. This type of exercise has gained popularity among males as well as women who want to bulk up physically. The most organic method to treat and respect your body is in this way.

Chapter 5

Living The Healthy Lifestyle

Knowing how to maintain your desired weight can help you avoid wasting all of your hard work once you've achieved it. When you reach the point where you have accomplished your weight loss target, the knowledge you have gained in advance will be helpful. You obviously want to keep up your newly discovered healthy lifestyle and would not want to mar the celebration you will want to have.

• **Don't skip any meals!** Remember, your body's metabolism will take this as a signal that your body is starving and will begin to store fat for reserves. Make sure you keep up with eating your meals, scheduled out as you have been. Besides, if you skip a meal at one point in the day, it could mean you overeat later on when you are just so hungry.

- **Keep eating a variety of foods.** This will help you to keep getting all the nutrients and vitamins your body needs to stay working properly. It will keep you feeling healthy, energized and protect your body by keeping it healthy. You can include choices from whole grains, fruits, vegetables and lean proteins.

- **Keep up the exercising!** Don't get lazy and slack off on your exercise routine now. You have gained the knowledge of what kind of a workout is right for you, and probably how to change it up every once in a while as well if you had instruction from a personal trainer.

Changing up your routine is a great idea to keep you from getting bored, and to keep your body guessing. As long as you are always combining your cardio and strength training, you will continue to stay fit and feel strong and healthy, all while protecting yourself further from illnesses coupled with your healthy diet.

- **Adjust your daily caloric intake.** Many

people ponder whether they should immediately boost their daily caloric intake. It is usually best to go gently, though. Start with just 250 extra calories per day. Check your weight once a week. Most likely, you still have some further weight to lose. If so, increase your calorie intake by another 250, then weigh yourself a week later. When you weigh yourself at the end of the week, keep going through these processes until you see that your weight has stayed the same. If you've gained a little weight, reduce it by 100 calories at a time until it stabilizes and stays the same from week to week.

• **Keep drinking that water!** Don't forget to have at least eight glasses of water a day to keep your body working well. Water aides in digestion, increases your energy and helps rid your body of toxins naturally. Plus, you will stay hydrated and healthy.

• **Keep eating frequently.** You have probably already figured out that eating five to six modest meals a day is a smart idea because it keeps your metabolism going and leaves you feeling satiated. It is crucial to keep doing this as well since, if this was an issue in the past, you don't want to fall into the trap of raising your portion sizes once more. One day you'll find yourself right back where you started. You will at the very least put on a lot of the weight you worked so hard to lose again.

- **Don't let the junk food back in.** Why destroy your new healthy routines by reverting to your old behaviours and overindulging in junk food? You've learned how to satisfy all of your cravings with delicious, nutritious foods. Maintain a daily diet of fruits and vegetables of at least six to eight servings.

- **Take your daily vitamins.** Do not stop taking your daily vitamin supplements. By doing this, you can ensure that you get all the vitamins you need each day and that you keep a healthy weight.

The Secrets of Staying Healthy

Nobody wants to assume they will contract a serious illness; everyone wants to enjoy long, healthy lives. There are measures to help safeguard ourselves that can help make our lives more full and healthy overall, even while we can't forecast or prevent every incident.

- **Prevention and early detection is the first thing you should consider.** A good doctor and making these visits will help you stay healthy because your doctor can spot things that you can't on your own. Most individuals dread getting their annual physicals or even going to the dentist every six months.

Knowing your family history is essential because your doctor can monitor your symptoms and perform routine tests if there is a history of cancer or heart disease in your family.

- **Love the people you are with.** Spend time with the people who are always there for you, such as your husband, kids, extended family, friends, and co-workers. Enjoy your interactions with others and uphold wholesome friendships. You need these connections in order to feel fulfilled in life.

- **Get eight hours of sleep.** Although many people find this one difficult to do because of how busy we can get in our lives, it really is very important to leading a happy and healthy life.

- **Find something you are good at.** All of us have times where we need to be doing something we really enjoy, and most of these are things that we excel at. This is usually something that makes us feel good inside as well, and can even be soothing and stress relieving.

- **Manage your stress – don't ignore it!** Everyone experiences some form of stress, and it's crucial that we manage it to prevent it from becoming overwhelming and taking over our lives.
You can actually become physically ill when

you are plagued by anxiety and stress in a number of ways. Daily walks can help you relax and ensure that you are not overloading your schedule with commitments or letting other people's schedules control your day.

• **Find balance in your life.** Don't try to take on too many projects at work or let work consume you. Find a balance so you are still able to enjoy all the other things around you like your hobbies and your friends and family.

Although financial times can be tough, it is still so very important to find time to spend at least with your family, the ones you are working so hard to keep safe and provided for.

The Advantages of Staying Healthy

The benefits of staying healthy are boundless. It doesn't just mean that you are happy with the way you look and can fit into that new outfit. Being healthy has to do with your whole physical, mental and social well-being.

• **Your Physical Health:** Keeping your body in good shape can benefit you in many ways. It not only enables you to participate in daily tasks like walking, moving, and bending, but it also gives you the physical capacity to look after your dependent family members.

If you avoid diseases that were preventable and that would be very expensive, it may be financially advantageous.

• **Disease Prevention:** Making sure you are eating a healthy diet is vital to your overall health and staying healthy. The foods you Your physical health will be impacted if your mental health is poor. Many people are unaware of the significance of their mental health to their general wellbeing. It can make you ill if you let yourself become overly worried or if that tension takes control of your life.

Your chance of having a heart attack or stroke increases if you are under stress. You must find healthy strategies to manage your stress, such as through exercise, meditation, or counselling. Avoid handling stress in bad ways, such as by smoking, drinking, or eating unhealthy foods .choose to eat can have a direct impact on your health.

Phytochemicals are crucial for your health and may help ward off conditions including high blood pressure, certain types of cancer, diabetes, and heart disease. Only specific foods, like berries, spinach, olives, and kale, contain them. Consume a low-fat diet rich in whole grains, fruits, and vegetables to help safeguard your cardiovascular health.

- **Long Life:** You may be able to live a long and healthy life if you make an effort to lead a healthy lifestyle. Although not all illnesses can be avoided
Although some of your problems are beyond your control, you may help to prevent many of the most important ones by leading a healthy lifestyle.
Chronic diseases including diabetes, heart disease, stroke, and cancer are the major causes of death. Making lifestyle choices

that include restricting your diet, maintaining a healthy weight, getting enough exercise, and managing your stress can greatly reduce your risk of developing these conditions.

Maintaining a healthy lifestyle can also lift your spirits, increase your sense of worth, and sharpen your mind. You will be more physically fit, have more endurance, and be able to sleep better at night.
Improved digestion and decreased blood pressure are two additional advantages of leading a healthy lifestyle. Maintaining good health can also help you reduce or completely get rid of back discomfort and difficulties, as well as improving your balance and coordination, posture, and resting heart rate.

Conclusion

Ready...Set...Go!

Now that we've learnt how to improve your lifestyle and lose weight now, everybody knows what to do. They read the information, they recognize they need to take action and put in the effort but the truth of the issue is, people seldom do. Unless you discipline yourself to resist the temptation of eating unhealthy foods and drive yourself to eat healthy foods, you will find it difficult to get on the path to a healthy life.

No amount of reading or declaring "Yes, I can do it" will help you unless you take that initial step. It takes a tremendous commitment to start on track and it needs an equally strong commitment to maintain at it. Most people abandon up after a short period since they're not satisfied with their achievements. If you can commit and keep yourself motivated and continue to aim to eat properly and train well, you will attain your objective. No matter what the goal is, be it to lose weight or build your endurance or become a better athlete in a specific sport, you just need to go out there and make the effort and do the work required.

Over the course of time, not only will you psychologically adjust to your workout regiment but you will build a great degree of discipline and self-confidence and you will automatically retain a positive attitude which means easily being able to resist any form of temptation. Everybody needs to start from someplace. Setting your goals little by little as opposed to attempting to go all-out and trying to sweat out 10 pounds on the treadmill in the course of a week would do more harm than good. Starting the process slowly is crucial which means going for a brisk walk to help acclimatize your body to the more demanding runs you plan to accomplish in the following weeks.

One error people make when starting out is going all out which leads to injury and soon they feel that training is simply too unpleasant and taxing. As previously, make a timetable and if necessary, consult with a personal trainer about what would be good for you if you feel uncomfortable coming up with a schedule. Although you do not need to make the process that complicated. If your objective is to lose weight, all you truly require is a little daily window devoted to your activity and keeping an eye on what you put in your body.

Simply be confident and work towards your goals. Be positive and you will obtain the outcomes you seek. As we approach Spring, maybe now is a good time to begin formulating that plan and implementing a course of action so you can get on the path to the great healthy lifestyle you deserve? ☐

www.ingramcontent.com/pod-product-compliance
Lightning Source LLC
Chambersburg PA
CBHW050252220526
45465CB00002B/656